Vegan Diet

50 Simple Vegetarian Recipes for Smart Vegans

(Fast & Easy Vegan Recipes for a Healthy Life)

Alton Hill

Published by Robert Satterfield Publishing House

© **Alton Hill**

All Rights Reserved

Vegan Diet Cookbook: 50 Simple Vegetarian Recipes for Smart Vegans (Fast & Easy Vegan Recipes for a Healthy Life)

ISBN 978-1-989682-98-2

All rights reserved. No part of this guide may be reproduced in any form without permission in writing from the publisher except in the case of brief quotations embodied in critical articles or reviews.

Legal & Disclaimer

The information contained in this book is not designed to replace or take the place of any form of medicine or professional medical advice. The information in this book has been provided for educational and entertainment purposes only.

The information contained in this book has been compiled from sources deemed reliable, and it is accurate to the best of the Author's knowledge; however, the Author cannot guarantee its accuracy and validity and cannot be held liable for any errors or omissions. Changes are periodically made to this book. You must consult your doctor or get professional medical advice before using any of the suggested remedies, techniques, or information in this book.

TABLE OF CONTENT

Part 1 1
Chapter 1: Breakfast 2
Breakfast Quinoa 2
Southwestern Tofu Scramble 3
Apple Spice Breakfast Lentils 5
Red Lentils & Oats Porridge 6
Peanut Butter Banana Breakfast Pizza 8
Savort Lentil + Quinoa Protein Pancakes 9
Vegan Protein Pancackes 12
Vegan Gluten Free Omlettes 13
Peanut Butter And Jelly Stuffed Pancakes 15
Scrambled Tofu Breakfast Wrap 18
Tofu Scrambled "Eggs" 19
Thick Banana Peanut Butter 20
Healthy Edamame Sweet Potato Hash 21
High Protein Vanilla Chia Pudding 23
Buckwheat Crepes + Chocolate Sauce............. 23
Chapter 2: Main Courses 26
Kale Salad With Chickpeas And Spicy Tempeh Bits............. 26
Teriyaki Tofu Burger 28
Mexican Style Protein Bowl 29
Black Bean Lentil Salad With Cumin-Lime Dressing.......... 32
Carrot Slaw With Smoky Maple Tempeh Triangles 34
Arugula Lentil Salad Supreme 37
Tofu Broccoli Salad... 38
Shine Salad 40
Avocado & White Bean Salad With Vinaigrette............... 41
The Ultimate Vegan Protein Burrito 43
Summertime Chili 46

- White Bean & Cashew Ricotta Roast 48
- Hummus & Avocado Sandwich 50
- Kale, Mushroom, And Edamame Bowl With Brown Rice . 55
- Meaty Vegan Mushroom And Tvp Meatballs.................... 58
- Best Ever Vegan Creamy Broccoli Cheese Soup 62
- Quick & Easy Warming Tomato And Lentil Stew.............. 66
- Protein Monster Vegan Enchiladas.................................. 68
- Protein Packed Vegan Sloppy Joes 71
- Baked Sriracha & Soy Sauce Tofu 73
- Simple Vegan Tofu Lasagna 79
- Chapter 3: Smoothies 82
- Coffee Cashew Smoothie 82
- Raspberry Walnut Smoothie 82
- Cinnamon Apple Smoothie.. 83
- Green Protein Power Breakfast Smoothie....................... 84
- Apple Spinach Protein Smoothie 85
- Cofee Cashew And Cacao Protein Smoothie 86
- Protein Frosty Shake... 87
- Chocolate Peanut Butter Protein Shake 88
- Cherry Almond Smoothie.. 89
- Blueberry Banana Protein Smoothie 90
- Cinnamon Apple Smoothie.. 91
- Chapter 4: Snacks 93
- Blueberry Lemon Protein Scones.................................... 93
- Loaded Blueberry Muffins 96
- Petite Vanilla Bean Scones 97
- Part 2 102
- Introduction 103
- Lemon Squares... 103
- Crust: 104
- Filling:... 104

KEY LIME PIE	105
VEGAN CHEESECAKE	106
CRUST:	106
FILLING:	107
VEGAN CHOCOLATE FUDGE BROWNIES	108
CHOCOLATE VEGAN CHEESECAKE	109
CHOCOLATE BANANA CAKE	111
CREAMY PEANUT BUTTER PIE	112
FILLING:	112
STRAWBERRY CHEESECAKE	113
LEMON BUNDT CAKE	114
CRANBERRY BANANA COOKIES	116
VEGAN VANILLA CAKE	117
CHOCOLATE CHIP COOKIES	118
CARROT CAKE	120
APPLESAUCE CRANBERRY CAKE	121
OATMEAL COOKIES	122
PEANUT BUTTER COOKIES	124
APPLE CAKE	125
COCONUT LEMON CAKE	126
CHOCOLATE CHIP PUMPKIN COOKIES	128
PUMPKIN CHEESECAKE	129
GINGERSNAP COOKIES	132
GREEN TEA COOKIES	133
PEANUT BUTTER BALLS	134
BANANA CAKE	135
APPLE SPICE COOKIES	136
EASY DATE BANANA COOKIES	138
SPICE CAKE	139
OATMEAL RAISIN COOKIES	140
VEGAN LEMON COOKIES	142

- Pecan Cheesecake 143
- Crust: 143
- Filling: 143
- Coconut Banana Cookies 144
- Lemon Cake 146
- Frosted Raspberry Chocolate Cake 147
- Frosting: 149
- Molasses Cookies 149
- About The Author 152

Part 1

Chapter 1: Breakfast

Breakfast Quinoa

Ingredients:

Washed raw quinoa - 1 cup

Water - 1 cup

Apricot nectar - 1 cup (or any other nectar without additional sugar)

Chopped apples - 2

Washed blueberries - 1 cup

Diced walnuts - 2 tablespoons

Daiya yogurt - 2 cups

Directions:
- Rinse Quinoa
- Place Quinoa in pot add water and nectar and bring to a boil.
- Reduce heat, and simmer while covered.
- Cook for about 10-15 minutes, until all liquid is absorbed.

- Remove from heat and allow to cool.
- When quinoa is completely cool, toss it with fruits like blueberries, diced apples, and add chopped walnuts.
- Serve with yogurt on top.

Southwestern Tofu Scramble

Ingredients:

Extra-firm tofu - 2 blocks (14-ounce)

Grape seed oil - 2 tablespoons

Diced onion - 1 small onion

Finely diced green bell pepper - 1 small

Finely diced red bell pepper - 1 small

Crushed coriander - 1/2 teaspoon

Crushed cumin - 1/2 teaspoon

Crushed turmeric - 1-1/2

Washed and sieved black beans - 1 can (15-ounce)

Roughly chopped fresh cilantro - 1/4 cup

Kosher salt, freshly ground pepper

Warmed whole wheat tortillas - 4-6

Garnishes: salsa, sliced avocado, crushed vegan cheddar, chopped scallions, and hot pepper sauce (optional)

Directions:
- Drain liquid from tofu by placing it over layers of paper towels on a plate.
- Smash tofu using a potato masher or fork.
- In a large skillet, heat oil over medium-high heat.
- Sautee onion and peppers, cook until softened, about 3-4 minutes.
- Mix in cumin and coriander and cook for about 1 minute or until fragrant.
- Fold in mashed tofu, then turmeric and beans.
- Continue to cook for 1-2 minutes, until heat is distributed through; while frequently stirring.
- Add in cilantro and season with salt and pepper to taste
- Can be served with tortillas and garnishes as preferred.

Apple Spice Breakfast Lentils

Ingredients:

Red lentils soaked for 4 hours - 1 cup (to enable easy digestion)

Red rooibos tea - 3 cups

Chopped apples - 2 cored

Crushed cinnamon - 1 tablespoon

Crushed cloves - 1 teaspoon

Crushed turmeric - 1 teaspoon (optional, but it is very good)

Maple syrup, to taste (I buy Trader Joe's or online for the best value)

So Delicious® Dairy Free Vanilla Coconut Milk- add to your taste

Pinch of cinnamon (optional)

Directions:
- Soak and drain lentils.
- In a pot, submerge lentils with brewed tea and bring to a boil.

- Once boiling, reduce to low-medium heat.
- Simmer for ten minutes.
- Add in diced apples and spices.
- Continue to cook until tender, about 30 to 40 minutes more.
- Makes 4 small servings of a half cup each.
- Serve in serving bowls and drizzle each with maple syrup and pour in a munificent amount of coconut milk.

Red Lentils & Oats Porridge

Ingredients:

Red lentils - ½ cup

Rolled oats - 1 cup (thick/jumbo rolled oats)

Turmeric powder - ½ teaspoon

Coriander powder - 1 teaspoon

Dried, frozen or fresh curry leaves - 4 - 5

Dried thyme or 2-3 sprigs fresh thyme - ½ teaspoon

Nutritional yeast - 1 tablespoon plus extra if needed

Defrosted peas - 2 - 3 tablespoons

Salt to taste

Directions:
- Wash and drain lentils in cold water repeatedly until water runs clear.
- In a saucepan, pour 1 ½ cups of water and add lentils.
- Cook covered on medium heat until softened, about 10 minutes.
- Move lid to cover the pan partially; if the water is boiling over.
- Frequently check water levels to monitor if the liquid is drying out. Most of it will be absorbed.
- Make space by clearing lentils off a small section of the saucepan.
- Add in coriander powder, turmeric, and curry leaves. The spices will release flavor as they touch the hot pan.
- For 10 seconds, lightly roast the spices and then mix it into the lentils.

- Fold in the rolled oats with 2 ½ cups of water.
- Stir in until completely mixed.
- Cook until the oats have cooked through, absorbing the liquid.
- Takes between 5 to 8 minutes to cook, depending on the type of oats used.
- Add water as required or to preferred creaminess or texture.
- Mix in peas, nutritional yeast, dried thyme.
- Season with salt to taste.
- Remove from heat and serve warm.

Peanut Butter Banana Breakfast Pizza

Ingredients:
For the crust:

Chickpea flour - ¼ cup

Almond milk - ¼ cup

Pure maple syrup - 2 teaspoons

Cinnamon - ½ teaspoon

Vanilla extract - ½ teaspoon

For the toppings:

Creamy peanut butter - 1-2 tablespoons

Chopped ripe banana 1

Any toppings you want (my toppings were hemp seeds and cacao nibs)

Drizzle of pure maple syrup

Directions:
- Spray oil in a medium skillet and place over medium heat.
- Meanwhile, whisk together the crust ingredients until smooth
- Pour crust batter into hot skillet and cook for 4-6 minutes, until firm enough then simply flip it.
- Flip to cook both sides until crust is set.
- Spread peanut butter, and top with banana slices.
- Drizzle with pure maple syrup.

Savort Lentil + Quinoa Protein Pancakes

Ingredients:
For the Pancakes

- Red lentils - 1 cup
- White quinoa - 1 cup
- Water - 1¼ cup
- Diced garlic - 1 clove
- Fresh cilantro leaves - ¼ cup
- Coconut oil - 1 tablespoon
- Fresh lemon juice - 1 tablespoon
- Apple cider vinegar - 1 tablespoon
- Baking powder - ¾ teaspoon
- Garlic powder - ½ teaspoon
- Coriander - ½ teaspoon
- Large grain sea salt - 1 to 1½ teaspoons
- Black pepper, to taste
- Seedless, veinless and diced serrano pepper - 1
- Diced shallots - 3 tablespoons

Toppings

- Chopped avocado
- Chopped cherry tomatoes
- Greens
- Creamy hemp seed and pepita dressing

Directions:
- Place lentils and quinoa into two separate airtight containers and fill with tap water enough to completely submerge contents.
- Keep at least 2 extra inches of water on top as liquids if you are to store it overnight.
- Refrigerate both containers for a minimum of 8 hours or overnight.
- Allow quinoa and lentils to drain, then rinse thoroughly.
- Using a food processor, mix lentils and quinoa with: coconut oil, 1 cup water, lemon juice, apple cider vinegar, cilantro leaves, minced garlic, baking powder, coriander, garlic powder, salt, and pepper.
- Blend completely smooth, about 2-3 minutes.
- Pour batter into a large mixing bowl and gently fold in the shallots and serrano peppers.

- Spray or Rub coconut oil in a medium skillet or griddle pan and place over medium heat.
- Drop a full scoop of batter into the hot skillet. Cook and flip for 2 to 7 minutes per side as each side turns a golden color.
- Repeat the same with the remaining batter.
- Makes 5-6 medium or 4 large pancakes.
- Serve warm and top with desired fresh vegetables.
- Leftovers can be stored and refrigerated.

Vegan Protein Pancackes

Ingredients:

Makes 8-10 large pancakes

Chickpea flour - 2/3 cup

Almond flour - 1/2 cup

Hemp protein powder - 2 teaspoons (optional)

A little salt

Baking powder - 2 teaspoons

Stevia - 1/2 packet or a few drops for sweetness

Almond milk - 1 1/4 cups

Flax meal - 1 tablespoon and warm water- 4 tablespoons

Directions:
- In a mixing bowl, mix flax meal with warm water, and set aside.
- On a separate bowl, mix together the flour, baking powder, salt, hemp, and stevia (if you are using dry stevia).
- Place skillet over medium heat, and allow to heat up.
- Whisk in almond milk and egg into the flax mixture, and slowly fold in dry ingredients.
- Scoop about ¼ cup pancake batter unto hot skillet.
- As bubbles start to form on top, gently flip them over, to cook both sides.
- Cook until brown.
  - Serve

Vegan Gluten Free Omlettes

Ingredients:

Firm silken tofu - 200g

Turmeric - ¼ teaspoon

Crushed garlic - ¼ teaspoon

Salt to taste (or for an "egg-like" flavor, you can use black salt (kala namak) it is sold in Indian grocery stores. It gives it an egg-like taste.

Nutritional yeast - 3 tablespoons

Soy milk - ¾ cup (or any vegan milk like cashew milk)

Tahini - 1 full teaspoon

White flour - 1 1/2 Tbsp white flour (it is better to use already mixed gluten free flour or you mix tapioca, rice and corn till you get the required amount).

Chickpea/gram flour - 1 tbsp

For the Filling:

Any vegan cheese of your choice - 4 slices, shaped into 2 inch squares

Oil for frying

Directions:
- In a metal or plastic mixing bowl, pour in all ingredients.
- Using an electric hand blender (or food processor) blend until all ingredients are combined in a smooth consistency.
- Heat a tiny amount of oil in a non-stick pan and allow to heat.
- Pour a scoop of the omelet batter into the hot pan.
- Allow a few seconds to set and then whirl the mixture around near the edge so that to distribute evenly.
- Shortly after a few seconds, place one slice of cheese (cut into small squares) and allow to melt.
- Using a spatula, gently work from the edge and flip one side to fold omelet half on top of itself.
- Flip the whole omelet to brown both sides.
- Serve with your choice of vegetables or vegan sausages with ketchup.

Peanut Butter and Jelly Stuffed Pancakes

Ingredients:
Almond milk - 1 cup

Apple cider vinegar - 1 teaspoon

Diced strawberries - 1 cup

Tapioca starch - ¼ teaspoon (optional)

White whole wheat flour, or whole wheat pastry flour -1 cup

Baking powder - 2 teaspoons

Flax meal - 1½ teaspoons

Salt - ¼ teaspoon

Peanut butter - 2 tablespoons

Coconut sugar - 1½ tablespoons

Grape seed oil, or melted coconut oil - 1 tablespoon and extra for cooking

Vanilla extract - 1 teaspoon

Directions:
- In a small bowl, mix almond milk and vinegar and set aside for 10 minutes.

- On a skillet or electric griddle, preheat 1 tsp of cooking oil over medium heat or at 350F.
- Meanwhile, using a microwave warm up strawberries, about 1 minute. Keep checking to ensure they do not bubble and spill over the bowl.
- Mash the strawberries, and if you are using Tapioca starch, add mix this in.
- In a mixing bowl, mix flax meal with salt, flour, and baking powder; Mix until thoroughly combined.
- Add in coconut sugar, peanut butter, vanilla and oil to milk mixture. Stir wet ingredients together.
- Gradually pour wet mixture into dry ingredients.
- Whisk ingredients together but avoid over-mixing, still allowing lumps to form.
- Set aside for 5 minutes.
- Scoop and pour 2 full tablespoons of pancake batter into the skillet or griddle.
- Allow to set and place about 1 tablespoon of mashed strawberries at the center of the pancake.
- Cover the strawberries with more batter.

- As the edges of the pancakes start to turn golden, flip to cook the other side.
- Follow cooking steps for the remaining dough.
- Serve pancakes with maple syrup or add peanut butter and strawberries for toppings.

Scrambled Tofu Breakfast Wrap

Ingredients:

1 recipe scrambled tofu

Whole grain wraps - 1 large wrap or 2 small wraps

Lettuce or baby spinach

Chopped tomato

Chopped avocado

Optional: hummus, sriracha, salsa or vegan mayo

Directions:
- Take a bed of lettuce and place it line down in the middle of a whole grain wrap.

- Place scrambled tofu, tomato, and avocado on top.
- You can try experimenting with different flavors by changing toppings or adding hummus, salsa, vegan mayo, sriracha, and other condiments.
- Bring the sides of the wrap together and fold.
- Hold together with a toothpick.
- NOTE:
- The scrambled tofu can be prepared and cooked in advance then reheated to assemble with your wrap.

Tofu Scrambled "Eggs"

Ingredients:

Organic sprouted firm tofu - 15 oz

Onion powder - ½ teaspoon

Garlic powder - ½ teaspoon

Sea salt - ¼ teaspoon

Turmeric powder - ¼ teaspoon

Vegetable stock - 3 tablespoons

Daiya vegan butter

Directions:
- Drain the tofu of its water.
- Place an ordinary nonstick skillet over medium-high heat.
- A regular skillet can be used, but ensure it is well-greased.
- You can also opt to grease a nonstick skillet with non-dairy butter for a creamier taste.
- Mix tofu and spices together.
- Using the edge of spatula, slice and dice the tofu while cooking in the pan to match scrambled eggs consistency.
- Slowly pour about 1 tablespoon vegetable broth at a time.
- Allow broth to boil each time so tofu can fully absorb it.
- Turn off heat and season with the dish with sea salt and pepper to taste.

Thick Banana Peanut Butter

Ingredients:
Diced frozen Bananas - 2

Small pitted Dates - 4 or Large pitted Medjool Dates- 2

Smooth Peanut Butter - 1 full tablespoon

Chia Seeds - 1 tablespoon

Hemp milk - 1/2 Cup (or any non-dairy milk)

Water for thinning the mixture - 1/4 Cup

Directions:
- Using a high-speed blender, blend all ingredients to make the puree.
- Blend until the puree has an entirely smooth consistency, and add water as needed.
- Set aside for about 3-5 minutes to allow the chia seeds to break down a tiny bit more. This will allow easier absorption of the nutrients they carry.

Healthy Edamame Sweet Potato Hash

Ingredients:
Olive oil - ½ tablespoon

Roughly diced red bell pepper - 1

Roughly diced shallot - 1 shallot

Boiled and minced sweet potato - 1 medium

Frozen edamame plus defrosted

salt & pepper - 2 cups

Garlic powder - ¼ teaspoon

Diced green onion

Directions::
- Heat olive oil in skillet
- Sautee shallot, bell pepper, and sweet potato on medium heat until cooked but crisp, around 3-5 minutes.
- Mix in the edamame and cook together for 3-4 minutes.
- Season the dish with salt, pepper, and garlic powder to taste.
- Mix in chopped green onion.
- Best served hot!
- NOTE:
- For faster cook time, precook sweet potato using a microwave for about 4-5 minutes or until fork-tender.

High Protein Vanilla Chia Pudding

Ingredients:

Boiled quinoa - ¼ cup

Chia seeds - 2 tablespoons

Hemp heart - 2 tablespoons

Vanilla powder - ¼ teaspoon

Little of stevia or 2 tablespoons maple syrup

Pinch of cinnamon

Cashew milk - ¾ cup cashew milk (or any vegan milk you prefer)

Directions:
- Stir together all ingredients in a jar.
- Seal with lid tightly.
- Refrigerate chia pudding and allow to set; this takes about 2 or more hours.
- Remove the pudding from the jar.
- Top with preferred toppings.

Buckwheat Crepes + Chocolate Sauce

Ingredients:

Crepes

Buckwheat flour - 1¼ cup

Rice flour - ½ cup

Arrowroot powder - 1 tablespoon

Rice or soy milk - 1 cup

Water - 1½ cup

Vanilla extract - 1 teaspoon

Sugar - 1 tablespoon

Ground flax seed - 1 tablespoon

Coconut oil to be used in the pan

Chocolate Sauce

Tahini - ½ cup (or any nut/seed butter)

Soy or almond milk - 3 tablespoons

Maple syrup - 2 tablespoons

Medjool dates - ½ cup

Cocoa powder - ¼ cup

Directions:

Crepes

- Preheat non-stick pan or a cast iron skillet over medium heat.
- Smear coconut oil on the pan just enough to grease it.
- Meanwhile, combine all ingredients into a blender, and process until smooth.
- Pour and spread the batter from the center of the hot skillet, allowing it to spread outward creating a thin layer forming the crepe.
- Allow to cook for about 4 minutes, then flip.
- Cook the other side for just around 2 minutes.
- In a folded, dry kitchen towel, place the crepe in the center and cover.
- Repeat cooking steps with the remaining batter.
- Crepes can be served with chocolate sauce (recipe below), toasted nuts, sliced fruit, and maple syrup.

Chocolate Sauce

- In a food processor, blend all ingredients until smooth.

Chapter 2: Main Courses

Kale Salad with Chickpeas and Spicy Tempeh Bits

Ingredients:
TEMPEH BITS:

Tempeh - 8oz

Vegetable oil - ¼ cup

Salt- ¼ teaspoon

Onion powder - 2 teaspoons

Garlic powder - 2 teaspoons

Sweet paprika - 2 teaspoons

Chili powder - 1 teaspoon

Lemon pepper - 1 teaspoon

Cayenne pepper - 1 teaspoon plus extra if you want it hot

Smoked sea salt (optional)

SALAD:

Diced kale - 1 lb.

Shredded carrots - 1 cup

Chick peas - 1 can (15.5oz)

Crispy sesame seeds - 2 cups

DRESSING:
Seasoned rice vinegar - 1 cup

Low sodium soy sauce - ¼ cup (Bragg liquid aminos can also be used)

Toasted sesame oil - 2 tablespoons

Freshly crushed ginger - 1 tablespoon

Directions:
- Add salt to boiling water.
- For 30 seconds, Soak kale in the boiling water.
- Rinse kale running under cold water and allow to drain.
- Once cooled, squeeze out any excess water and set aside.
- Set oven to 425F to preheat.
- In a little bowl, mix all spices for tempeh together.
- In another minute bowl, pour vegetable oil.
- Slice the tempeh into thin pieces.

- Take each slice and dip in vegetable oil.
- Line a baking sheet with parchment paper.
- Arrange tempeh slices on the baking sheet and sprinkle spices on top ensuring the open side if adequately covered.
- Bake for 20minutes at 425F, or until the slices show a golden brown color and are crispy (constantly check on them as they bake to keep them from burning).
- If you are using smoked sea salt, sprinkle this after cooking.
- In a large bowl, mix all salad ingredients.
- In a glass jar, combine and stir all dressing ingredients, shake well with the lid closed.
- Pour the salad dressing all over the salad and toss all ingredients to coat.
- Top with crumbled Tempeh on the top right before serving.

Teriyaki Tofu Burger

Ingredients:
Extra-firm tofu - 2 (3 oz)

Vegan Teriyaki marinade - 1 tablespoon

Sriracha - 1 tablespoon

Red chili flakes - 1 teaspoon

Chopped red onion - 1/4

Shredded carrot - 2 tablespoons

Butter leaf lettuce (to garnish)

Flat Out sandwich wraps

Directions:
- Prepare and heat the grill.
- Mix red chili flakes, teriyaki marinade, and Sriracha, and marinate tofu in this mixture.
- In a pan, caramelize red onions.
- Grill marinated tofu for about 3-4 min per side.
- Put grilled tofu on a flat out wrap.
- Top wrap with shredded carrots, butter leaf lettuce, and caramelized red onion.

Mexican Style Protein Bowl

Ingredients:

Boiled brown rice - 1/2 cup

Boiled Black Beans - 1/3 cup

Salsa - 2 full spoons

Diced Avocado - 1/4

Optional Add-ins

Plain Fat-free Greek Yogurt - 2 tablespoons

Hot Sauce of your choice

Directions:
Combine and Toss all ingredients in a bowl.

Tofu Bento

Ingredients:

Extra-firm Tofu - 1 packet

Boiled Brown Rice - 2 cups

Low-sodium Soy Sauce - 2 tablespoons

Ginger, Garlic Powder, and Onion Powder - 1 teaspoon each

Chili Paste - 1 teaspoon

Diced Broccolini - 1 bunch

Diced Red Bell Pepper - 1

Chopped Orange Bell Pepper - 1

Chopped Green Onion – 1/4 cup (optional)

Sriracha to top (optional)

Directions:
- Unpack tofu and drain excess moisture by pressing it with paper towels.
- Chop the tofu into small cube shapes and put inside a large Ziploc bag.
- Over medium heat, heat olive oil in a large saute pan.
- Stir-fry bell pepper and broccolini until lightly tender.
- On a separate pan, add tofu and stir-fry over medium heat for about 5 minutes, occasionally stirring until all edges turn a light brown.
- Serve with 1/2 cup of brown rice and add veggies, tofu, and green onions for toppings.

Black Bean Lentil Salad with Cumin-lime Dressing

Ingredients:

Green or brown dry lentils - 1 cup

Washed and sieved black beans - 15 oz. can

Red bell pepper - 1

Red onion - 1/2 small

Roma tomatoes - 1-2

Stemless, large bunch cilantro

Optional: green onion

{For the dressing}

Lime juice - 1 lime

Olive oil - 2 tablespoons

Dijon mustard - 1 teaspoon

Crushed garlic - 1-2 cloves

Cumin - 1 teaspoon

Oregano - 1/2 teaspoon

Salt - 1/8 teaspoon

Optional: chipotle powder, chili powder, pepper, hot sauce, other seasonings, etc.

Directions:

- Following package cooking instructions, cook lentils. This should leave it firm and not mushy.
- Drain lentils after cooking.
- Meanwhile, as lentils are cooking, prepare the dressing.
- In a small bowl, mix and combine all dressing ingredients and set aside.
- Dice the bell onion, pepper, and tomatoes finely. Moreover, chop the cilantro roughly.
- In a separate big bowl, Mix and toss the bell pepper, black beans, onion, lentils, and tomatoes.
- Mix in dressing and toss ingredients to coat.
- Lightly toss in cilantro.
- Serve right away or allow flavors to sip in by chilling covered for at least an hour in the fridge.

Carrot Slaw with Smoky Maple Tempeh Triangles

Ingredients:

Tempeh, shaped into triangles - 8 ounces

Liquid smoke - 1/4 teaspoon (optional)

Grade B maple syrup – 1 **1/2** Tablespoon

Extra virgin olive oil/virgin coconut oil - 1 teaspoon

Tamari- 2-3 teaspoons or soy sauce - 2 teaspoons

Grinded raw walnuts - 1 Tablespoon

Shredded carrots - 4 cups

Chopped onion - 1 small

Curry powder - 1 tablespoon

Tumeric powder - 1/4 teaspoon (optional)

Black pepper - 1/8 teaspoon

Tahini - 2 Tablespoon

Fresh lemon juice - 1/4 cup

Sweet stuff: Maple syrup- 1 - 1 1/2 Tablespoon and an handful of raisins (optional)

Finely diced flat leaf parsley - 1/2 cup and extra for garnishing

A few pinches of cayenne for heat (optional)

Salt and pepper for carrot salad - to taste

Black Bean Lentil Salad with Cumin Lime Dressing

Directions:
- Heat coconut oil or olive oil in a warm a skillet over high heat.
- Once the oil is hot, add the tamari, tempeh triangles, liquid smoke, and maple.
- Lightly toss the tempeh around as you cook to allow liquid to be absorbed.
- Cook tempeh for around 5 minutes, while constantly tossing the tempeh around.
- When you see the tempeh turning a brown color and edges turn a bit black,

while all liquid has dried up, remove it from the heat.
- Sprinkle the some black pepper and walnut pieces on top of the dish,
- Set the skillet aside, keeping the triangles warm in the pan.
- Meanwhile, in a big mixing bowl, mix the tahini, carrots, spices, lemon juice, parsley, onion, maple syrup, and optional raisins.
- Toss ingredients very well for a minute or 2 to allow the carrots to marinate in the dressing.
- Add a spoonful of tahini if you'd like to opt for a creamier salad
- For thinner and zestier taste, add a teaspoon of apple cider vinegar or another splatter of lemon juice.
- Finish the carrot salad by seasoning with salt and pepper to taste.
- In a large serving bowl, pour in the carrot salad with the tempeh on top.
- Serve directly or refrigerate for few hours to a day to allow the carrots to soften.

Arugula Lentil Salad Supreme

Ingredients:

Cashew nuts - 100g (about 1 cup)

Onion - 1

Olive oil - 3 tablespoons

Chilli/jalapeño - 1

Dried tomatoes - 5-6

Whole wheat bread - 3 slices

Lentils - 1 big can (15oz or 400g) boil before use

Aragula - 100g

Salt and pepper to taste

Optional: raisins, honey/agave nectar, lemon juice or vinegar

Directions:
- Using a pan on low heat, roast the cashews for around three minutes to make bring out the best of its aroma.
- Toss roasted cashews into the salad bowl.

- Finely dice the onion.
- Sautee, the onion in a pan, using a little oil for about 3 minutes on low heat.
- Chop the dried tomatoes and jalapeño/chili.
- Cut enlarged sized croutons out of the bread.
- Using the remaining oil, fry the crouton pieces in a pan until crispy.
- Season with salt and pepper to taste.
- Meanwhile, rinse the arugula and toss it into the bowl.
- Add the lentils in, and mix all ingredients together.
- Season with salt and pepper to taste.
- Serve with the croutons on top.

Tofu Broccoli Salad

Ingredients:

Broccoli - 1 head

Firm tofu - 4 oz

Nicely diced garlic - 1 clove

Minced green onion -1

Korean soy sauce -2 teaspoons for soup

Sesame oil - 1 teaspoon

Roasted sesame seeds - 2 teaspoons

Salt to taste if you wish

Directions:
- Slice broccoli florets into little pieces.
- Using a steamer, steam broccoli and tofu over medium heat for 2-3 minutes or just until the broccoli is green but tender.
- Remove broccoli from steamer and rinse in cold water.
- Put broccoli in a big shallow mixing bowl, and set aside.
- Place tofu inside a fine cotton cloth (or cheesecloth), wrap it to squeeze out excess water.
- Crush the tofu to crumbs and place beside broccoli without mixing yet.
- Add in green onion, garlic, 1 tsp of Korean soy sauce and massage onto the crumbled tofu alone. Seasoning just the tofu.

- Lightly pour the remaining 1 tsp soy sauce, sesame seeds and sesame oil over both the broccoli and tofu.
- Very lightly and gently toss all together.
- Season with salt to taste.
- Serve chilled or at immediately.

Shine Salad

Ingredients:

Sieved and washed Garbanzo Beans - 1 can (15oz)

Boiled Quinoa - 2 cups

Fine Extra Virgin Olive Oil - 2 tablespoons

White Wine Vinegar - 1 tablespoon

Agave Nectar - 1 teaspoon

Salt - 1/4 teaspoon

Diced Tomatoes - 1 cup

Sliced Cucumbers - 1 cup

Mixed Greens - 2 big handfuls

Sunflower Kernels - 1 tablespoon

Directions:
- Combine quinoa, garbanzo beans, vinegar, olive oil, agave nectar, and salt in a large bowl.
- Mix in remaining ingredients right before serving to eat.
- For advanced preparations, remaining ingredients must be stored separately.
- For a hint of spiciness, you can opt to sprinkle crushed red pepper or freshly cracked black pepper.
- You can choose to add in or use whatever vegetables available.
- Notes
- *Cook Quinoa following package instructions.
- *It is ideal to use the very best olive oil for this salad as it carries the most of the flavor. Olive oil that is more yellow than green seems to taste better, though without any scientific reason.

Avocado & White Bean Salad With

Vinaigrette

Ingredients:

- White beans - 1 can

- Sliced avocado - 1

- Diced Roma tomato - 1

- Minced sweet onion - 1/4 if you desire but you can forego it if you do not like onions

The above is used for the salad. Below is for the vinaigrette:

- Olive oil - 1 1/2 tablespoons

- Lemon juice - 1/4 cup

- Basil- Fresh or dried depending on your choice

- Minced garlic - a little (not too much to avoid overspicing)

- Salt & pepper to taste

- Mustard - 1 teaspoon

Directions:
- After completing the salad base prepare the vinaigrette next:

- Whisk together vinaigrette ingredients and pour over salad base
- Toss well to coat.
- Chill in the fridge for a couple of hours before serving.

The Ultimate Vegan Protein Burrito

Ingredients:
For the Quinoa
Well washed white quinoa- ¾ cup

Water- 1½ cups

Sea salt- ¼ teaspoon

Sieved and washed black beans- 1 can

Minced fresh cilantro- ¼ cup

Squeezed lime- 3 tablespoons

Hemp seeds- 3 tablespoons

Sea salt- ¼-1/2 teaspoon

black pepper to taste

For Kale
Stemless, diced kale- 3 cups

Squeezed lime- 1 tablespoon

Olive oil- ½ tablespoon

sea salt to taste

black pepper to taste

For the Pico de Gallo
1 cup of ¼ cleaved cherry tomatoes

Chopped red onion- ¼ cup

Diced cilantro- 2 tablespoons

sea salt to taste

For the Guacamole
Pitted avocado- 1

Squeezed lime- 1

sea salt for taste

Extra Ingredients

4 big germinated grain or grainless tortillas

Directions:

Quinoa Cooking Instructions

- Using a small pot, boil quinoa in water with ¼ teaspoon sea salt over medium-high.
- Lower heat once boiling and simmer while covered for 10-14 minutes, or just until quinoa is soft and translucent.
- Using a fork, fluff it around and pour it into a large bowl.
- Stir in the chopped cilantro, black beans, hemp seeds, lime juice, sea salt, and black pepper to the quinoa. Set aside.

For the Kale
- Chop kale and place in a bowl.
- Mix in olive oil, lime juice, and sea salt and massage into the kale for 2-3 minutes or until softened. Set this aside.

For the Pico de Gallo.
- In another bowl, mix red onion, cherry tomatoes, cilantro, and sea salt. Set aside.

For the Guacamole

- In a small bowl, combine the scooped out flesh of the avocado, juice from one lime and season with sea salt, to taste.
- Using a fork, mash the avocado to your desired consistency for the guacamole. Set aside.

To Assemble the Burritos
- On a clean surface, lay one tortilla flat.
- Fill the tortilla with the prepared quinoa mixture, kale, Pico de gallo, and guacamole.
- Roll the tortilla away from you into a burrito, tucking in the sides as you roll.
- Slice in the burrito in half and serve right away. Repeat to make more.
- Separately chill/refrigerate any leftover.

Summertime Chili

Ingredients:

Virgin olive oil- 2 tablespoons

Diced white onion- 1 cup

Chopped garlic- 2 cloves

Diced carrots- 2 carrots

Minced celery- 1 stalk celery

Diced zucchini- 1 cup

Minced summer squash- 1 cup

Diced red bell pepper- ½ pepper

Chili powder- 1½ tablespoons

Cumin- 1 teaspoon

Oregano- 1 teaspoon

Sea salt- ½ teaspoon

Cayenne pepper- ½ -1/4 teaspoon

Mashed tomatoes- 3 cups

Vegetable stock- 3 cups

Sieved and washed black beans- 1 can

Sieved and washed kidney beans- 1 can

Frosted corn- ½ cup

Directions:
- In a Dutch oven or large saucepan and heat olive oil over medium heat.
- Sautee onion until translucent, while constantly stirring.
- Add in garlic and Sautee with the onion until fragrant.

- Mix in celery, carrots, summer squash, zucchini, and bell pepper, and stir-fry ingredients until tender.
- Add crushed tomatoes, broth and seasonings then bring to a boil
- Once boiling, reduce heat to a low simmer.
- Mix in beans, and cook while partially covered
- Continue simmering for 30-45 minutes.
- Add in corn.
- Season to taste.

White Bean & Cashew Ricotta Roast

Ingredients:

Fresh cashew pieces (unroasted)- ½ cup

Hot tap water- ½ cup

Thoroughly sieved and washed cannellini or navy beans- 1 can (16-ounce)

Light-flavored olive oil- 2 teaspoons

Freshly juiced lemon- 2 teaspoons

Agave nectar- ½ teaspoon

Salt-½ teaspoon

Hot whole-grain or sourdough toast

SAVORY GARNISHES

Baby kale leaves

Cherry tomatoes, chopped

Sweet paprika, crushed

Black pepper, freshly crushed

SWEET GARNISHES

Strawberries, finely cut

Date syrup or unrefined maple syrup

Fresh mint leaves

Pink sea salt

Directions:

• In a small bowl, submerge the cashew pieces in hot water and keep soaked for a minimum of 20 minutes, or until the cashews are softened.

• Set aside 1 tablespoon of the water used for soaking.

- Drain away remaining liquid from cashews.
- Using a food processor, blend the softened cashews together with the left soaking water into thick, slightly grainy and pasty consistency.
- Mix in the olive oil, beans, agave nectar, lemon juice, and salt.
- Pulse in blender until mixture is thick. Stop occasionally to scrape down any ingredients on the sides of the bowl to ensure all is blended.
- Avoid over-blending; a grainy texture is preferable.
- Taste and season with a pinch of salt, lemon juice or sugar, to your desired taste.
- Enjoy right away or refrigerate for at least 30 minutes to allow flavors to develop.
- Slather the spread on hot toast and top with your choice of sweet or savory garnishes.

Hummus & Avocado Sandwich

Ingredients:

Sliced avocado- 1/2

Ezekiel sprouted grain bread- 2 slices

Hummus – that can be spread thickly on the two slices of bread (you can make yours or buy any organic flavored one you like from the store)

Tomato- 2 slices

Chopped cilantro- a pinch

Juiced lemon- 1 slice

Hot sauce, sprinkled

Sea salt to taste

Black pepper to taste

Directions:
- Toast bread slices to your desired consistency.
- Slather hummus on both slices of bread.
- Lay sliced avocado pieces and thinly sliced tomato slices on the bread
- Sprinkle cilantro on top.
- Squeeze out lemon juice around top.
- Sprinkle sea salt & pepper to taste.

- Drizzle with hot sauce.
- Place both slices together to close sandwich.
- Enjoy!

Vegan Chili

Ingredients:

Very mild olive oil- 1 tablespoon

Small onion- 1

Garlic- 2 cloves

Red bell pepper- 1

Cultivated jalapeno pepper- 1

Tvp-textured vegetable protein (2 tablespoons warm vegetable stock & 1 tablespoon low sodium soy sauce added to it)- 1 cup

Sodium-free chopped tomatoes (like Hunts chopped without salt)-1 can(15oz)

Low sodium vegetable stock-1½ cup low

Tomato paste- 1 cup

Hot sauce (for example cholula)- 1 tablespoon

Red wine- 1 tablespoon

Chili powder- 1 tablespoon

Smoked paprika- 1 teaspoon

Crushed cumin- ½ teaspoon

Dried thyme- ½ teaspoon

Dried oregano- ½ teaspoon

Himalayan or sea salt- ½ teaspoon

Crushed pepper for sprinkling

Cayenne pepper for flavor (optional)- 1 teaspoon

Sieved and washed red kidney beans- 1 can (15oz)

Sieved and washed black beans, pinto beans or cannellini beans-1 can (15oz)

GARNISH

Cilantro/parsley leaves, little quantity

Crushed pepper to sprinkle

Directions:
- Dice onion finely into small cubes.
- Finely chop garlic into small pieces.

- Heat 1 tablespoon extra light olive oil in a medium saucepan over medium-high heat.
- Sautee onions and garlic until browned.
- Separately, cut the bell pepper in small square pieces.
- Then cut the jalapeno pepper open in half allowing you to remove the seeds and middle inner stem, then chop it into tiny cubes.
- In a small bowl, place the TVP.
- In a separate bowl, mix broth and soy sauce, then heat it up.
- Drizzle the soy sauce and broth mixture on the TVP and allow it to hydrate. Set aside.
- After onions have been browned and cooked for about 10 minutes, toss in the jalapeno and red pepper. Stir-fry for about 3 minutes.
- Add the minced and hydrated TVP and continue to cook while stirring for another 3 minutes.
- As this cooks, drain two cans of beans from liquid and thoroughly rinse them well, and drain again of all excess liquid.

- Mix in the waiting ingredients. This includes the vegetable broth, the can of diced tomatoes, blazing sauce, chili powder, red wine, cumin, smoked paprika, oregano, thyme, cayenne(if using for spice), salt, and pepper.
- Mix the finally add in the beans.
- Cooked covered and reduce heat to a simmer and cook for about 25 minutes, continuously stirring every 5 minutes.
- Garnish and prepare the dish with whole/chopped cilantro or parsley leaves and sprinkle with some pepper.

Kale, Mushroom, and Edamame Bowl with Brown Rice

Ingredients:

Cooked brown rice

Veggies

Very mild olive oil- 1 tablespoon

Medium onion- ½

Garlic- 2 cloves

Himalayan/sea salt- a pinch, small

Fresh shiitake mushrooms- 6

Tvp-textured vegetable protein- 2 tablespoons (add 1 tablespoon hot water)

Celery- 2 stalks

Iced edamame beans- ½ cup

Water- ½ cup & 2 tablespoons

Cooking wine, white- 2 tablespoons

Cornstarch- 1 tablespoon

Low sodium soy gravy- 1 teaspoon

Sesame oil- 1 teaspoon

Himalayan or sea salt- ½ teaspoon

Crushed ginger- 1 teaspoon

Crushed pepper for sprinkling

Kale- a big handful

Directions:
- Finely dice the onions into tiny cubes
- Finely chop the garlic into small pieces.
- Heat 1 tablespoon of olive oil with a little pinch of salt in a saucepan over high heat

- Sautee the onions and garlic until browned, about 12 minutes, continually stirring to keep from burning any sides
- Meanwhile, prepare shitake mushrooms by removing the stems and slicing them thinly.
- In a small bowl, place the TVP and stir in a tablespoon of hot tap water. Mix it around and allow a few minutes ; this to rehydrate.
- After sauteing the onions for 12 minutes, add the mushrooms and TVP. Stir and cook for about 3 minutes.
- Separately, finely dice celery into tiny cubes.
- Prepare edamame beans read.
- After 3 minutes, Stir-fry celery and edamame seeds together with the garlic and onion. Cook for together for 3 more minutes.
- Meanwhile, combine the water, cornstarch, white wine/white cooking wine, sesame oil, ground ginger, soy sauce, salt, and ground pepper together.

- Continue to mix and stir until dry ingredients have completely dissolved into the liquid.
- Pour this into the saucepan after cooking the celery and edamame for 3 minutes.
- Stir around for a second, then directly add a big handful of kale.
- Continue to cook for final 4-5 minutes while constantly stirring.
- Remove from heat once ingredients have mixed evenly and kale is tender (but still has a vibrant green color).
- To Serve: Scoop brown rice into a serving bowl, about half filled, add veggies for toppings.

Meaty Vegan Mushroom and TVP Meatballs

Ingredients:

Fresh shiitake mushrooms- 4 cups

Cremini mushrooms- 2 cups

Medium yellow onion- ½ or 1 small yellow onion

Garlic- 2 cloves

Extra virgin olive oil- ¼ teaspoon

Low sodium soy gravy- 1 tablespoon

Sesame oil- 1 teaspoon

Ground fennel seeds- 1 teaspoon

Onion powder- 1 teaspoon

Garlic powder- 1 teaspoon

Smoked paprika- 1 teaspoon

Chipotle pepper- ½ teaspoon

Crushed mustard- ½ teaspoon

Red pepper flakes- a pinch

Himalayan/sea salt- a little pinch

Tvp-textured vegetable protein- ½ cup (add 3 tablespoons of hot water)

Vital wheat gluten- ½ cup

Corn or tapioca starch- 1 tablespoon

Sesame oil- 1 tablespoon

Low sodium soy sauce- 1 teaspoon

Garlic powder- 1 teaspoon

Smoked paprika- 1 teaspoon

Himalayan or sea salt- ¼ teaspoon

Cayenne pepper- 1 teaspoon

Crushed pepper for sprinkling

Directions:

• Prepare oven and preheat to 275°F (135°C).

• Finely chop the shiitake mushrooms (using the Asian huagu, a shiitake mushroom with a large flower shape on its top, is ideal, but regular shitake mushrooms will do)

• Thinly slice cremini mushrooms into thick pieces.

• Peel and dice onion into tiny cubes.

• Finely chop garlic into small pieces

• Combine chopped ingredients in a large bowl.

• Drizzle in olive oil, sesame oil, soy sauce, and add in hand-crushed fennel seeds, garlic powder, onion powder, paprika, mustard, chipotle pepper, red pepper flakes and salt.

• Using your hands, massage all ingredients into the mushrooms until the

sauce is evenly coating and absorbed by the mushrooms, garlic, and onion
- Prepare a 9×13 inch rectangular baking tray and spray it with non-stick cooking oil
- Arrange and spread the mushrooms on the tray.
- Bake for 20 minutes at 275°F (135°C).
- This will soften the mushrooms a lot.
- Place baked mushrooms in a food processor (or blender, but avoid using high powered blenders) and blend until the mushrooms show a finely minced consistency.
- Transfer it to a large bowl.
- Meanwhile, mix 3 tablespoons of hot tap water with half a cup of TVP
- Stir until TVP is softened.
- Add softened TVP to the bowl of mushroom mince
- Mix in vital corn/tapioca starch, wheat gluten, soy sauce, sesame oil, paprika, garlic powder, salt, cayenne pepper and ground pepper.
- Continue to stir until ingredients are evenly and well mixed.

- Turn up the heat of the oven to 300°F (148°C).
- Clean the same baking tray used and spray again with nonstick cooking oil
- Roll the prepared mixture into palm sized balls and arrange them on the oven tray.
- Generously spray top of the balls with non-stick cooking oil,
- Bake for one hour
- Allow to cool and serve with Rao's Arrabbiata or with pasta.

Best Ever Vegan Creamy Broccoli Cheese Soup

Ingredients:

Extra virgin olive oil- 1 tablespoon

Nicely chopped large yellow onion- about 1½ cups

Diced medium shallot- 1

Smoked paprika- 1 teaspoon

Sea salt to taste- 2 teaspoons split and extra to taste

Black pepper, crushed, to taste

Stemless broccoli- 4 small or 2 big heads diced into bits of ½-inch florets (you need about 5 to 6 cups or a pound of florets)

Low-sodium vegetable stock- 4 cups

Distilled water- 2 cups

Small cauliflower florets- 2 cups

Manitoba Harvest Hemp Hearts- ½ cup (peeled hemp seeds)

Skinned, diced and roasted red peppers- ½ cup (you can use roasted red peppers in jars)

Nutritional yeast- ½ cup

Arrowroot powder- 1 tablespoon

Apple cider vinegar- 1 tablespoon

Freshly squeezed lemon juice -1 tablespoon (to mix the flavors and give them a pop sound)

Low sodium tamari for deep flavoring- 1 tablespoon

Directions:

- Using a stock pot or large dutch oven, heat up the olive oil over medium-low.
- Add and sauté the shallot, onion, smoked paprika, 1 tsp sea salt, and black pepper,
- Sauté until the onion is tender and translucent, about 6 minutes. Stir occasionally.
- Add 3 cups of the vegetable broth, filtered water, and the broccoli florets
- Bring up the temperature to medium-high, allow to a quick simmer for about 5 minutes.
- Lower heat to medium-low, and simmer covered for about 20 to 25 minutes or just until you find the broccoli florets have become fork-tender,
- Stir often to make sure that the broccoli is immersed in the liquids.
- Meanwhile, boil water in a medium pot. Add in the cauliflower florets into this pot and allow to boil until softened or fork-tender, about 7 minutes. Remove from heat and drain excess water.
- Take the cooked cauliflower florets, and add this to along with the Hemp Hearts,

nutritional yeast, arrowroot powder, remaining 1 cup of vegetable broth, apple cider vinegar, roasted red peppers, and the remaining 1 teaspoon of sea salt to a high-speed blender.
- Pulse on high for about 2 minutes or until the mixture has a completely smooth and creamy. This makes the "cheddar" sauce
- Pour the cauliflower "cheddar" sauce into the pot.
- Fold in and stir to combine.
- Bring up the temperature to medium and while continuously stirring for 3 to 5 minutes or until the broth thickens slightly. Avoid overheating so the arrowroot does not lose its thickening power.
- As soon as the broth has slightly thickened, turn off the heat and mix in the tamari and fresh lemon juice.
- Taste test and season it with more sea salt, black pepper, and smoked paprika, to your liking. (Some prefer to add another ½ teaspoon sea salt, and a few sprinkles of

freshly ground black pepper, and a few pinches of smoked paprika.)
- This dish can be enjoyed as soup or can be blended further as a puree to your preferred texture.
- Serve in bowls, sprinkle with new Hemp Hearts (if preferred)
- Keep leftovers in the fridge.

Quick & Easy Warming Tomato And Lentil Stew

Ingredients:

Extra-virgin olive oil- 2 tablespoons

Skinned and chopped yellow onion- 1 medium

Chopped garlic- 2 cloves

Dried rosemary- 1½ teaspoons

Sea salt- 1 teaspoon

Ground red pepper flakes- ¼ teaspoon or enough for desired taste

Raw, washed and sorted french green lentils- 1 cup

Crushed tomatoes without salt- 1 can (28-ounce)

Distilled water- 2 cups

Low sodium tamari- 1½ tablespoons

Balsamic vinegar- 2 tablespoons

Fresh thyme- 2 sprigs

Directions:
- In a large stock pot or dutch oven, heat olive oil over medium heat.
- Add in the onion and stir-fry until soft and translucent, about 6 minutes
- Add the chopped garlic, the dried rosemary, sea salt, and the red pepper flakes. Allow to cook together for another 1 to 2 minutes or just until the garlic is softened. Cook while stirring often.
- Mix in the filtered water, crushed tomatoes, french lentils, tamari, and balsamic.
- Stir continuously to combine flavors and let the sprigs of thyme settle into the broth.

- Bring up the temperature to medium-high and bring it to a quick boil.
- As soon as boiling, turn down heat to low, and simmer while covered for 30 to 35 minutes or until the lentils have become tender.
- Cautiously remove the thyme sprigs from the broth.
- Season with sea salt to taste.

Protein Monster Vegan Enchiladas

Ingredients:

Onion- 1

Red bell pepper- 1

Black beans- 15 oz. can

Garbanzo beans- 15 oz. can

Hemp hearts- 1/2 cup

Nutritional yeast- 1/3 cup

Roma tomatoes- 3

Cumin-2 teaspoons

Smoked paprika- 1 teaspoon

Salt to taste

Big tortillas- 6

Extras: spinach, chipotle, garlic

{For the enchilada sauce}

Organic low sodium vegetable stock- 3 cups

Tomato paste- 1/4 cup

All-purpose or no gluten flour- 1/4 cup

Olive oil- 2 Tablespoon

Cumin- 2 teaspoon

Chili powder- 1/2 teaspoon

Garlic powder- 1/4 teaspoon

Onion powder-1/4 teaspoon

Salt/pepper

Extras: cayenne pepper, crushed chipotle, smoked paprika, etc.

Directions:
- Finely dice the onion and bell pepper.
- Using a large skillet stir-fry onion and bell pepper for 8 minutes over medium heat.

- Meanwhile, cube tomatoes into small pieces and rinse beans in water.
- Once onions have become tender; lower heat and add in paprika, cumin, tomatoes, hemp hearts, nutritional yeast, garbanzo and black beans. Mix well.
- Allow to cook for 4-5 minutes. Set aside.
- Bake the Enchilada:
- Prepare and preheat the oven to 350F.
- Use a 9x13 baking dish lightly sprayed with olive oil
- Cover the bottom of the baking dish with 1 layer of enchilada sauce.
- Place the bean mixture in the middle of the tortillas. Roll up tortilla, and tuck in both ends.
- Place them in the baking dish and pour the remaining sauce on top.
- Bake at 350F for about 25 minutes.
- Serve with cilantro, avocado, hemp hearts, and nutritional yeast as desired for toppings.
- Instructions for Enchilada sauce:
- In a small mixing bowl, mix flour and spices together.

- Heat olive oil in a medium saucepan over medium heat.
- Once the oil is hot, slowly add tomato paste, cumin, flour, garlic powder, onion powder, and chili powder.
- Cook about 1 minute while continuously whisking.
- Pour in the broth and mix well with a whisk.
- Increase the temperature to it bring to a light boil.
- Reduce heat to a simmer and allow to cook for 8 minutes more, while whisking occasionally.
- Season with salt to taste.

Protein packed Vegan Sloppy Joes

Ingredients:

Black dry lentils- 1 cup

Dry quinoa- ½ cup

Vegetable stock for boiling- ½ cup

Water- 3 cups or more as needed

Diced onion- 1 medium

Sliced carrots- 2 large carrots

Diced red or green pepper- ½

Minced garlic- 3 cloves

Tomato sauce- 1 can (8 ounce)

Brown sugar- 2 tablespoons

Yellow mustard- 1½ tablespoons

Vegan Worcestershire sauce- 1 tablespoon

Apple cider vinegar- 2 tablespoons

Hot sauce- ½ tablespoon or more as desired

Paprika- 1 teaspoon

Salt- 1 teaspoon

Crushed black pepper to taste

Hamburger buns- 8

Directions:
- Using a small saucepan, combine the water, lentils, and salt.
- Boil lentils over high heat, then reduce temperature to a simmer. Cook for about 20 minutes, or until the lentils become tender. Drain excess water and set aside.

- Heat oil in a medium saucepan over medium-low heat.
- Stir-fry the onions and garlic for a few minutes.
- Add in cumin and chili powder
- Continue to cook until spices are fragrant, about a few minutes
- Add in the remaining ingredients, including boiled lentils (except buns of course)
- Continue to simmer while occasionally stirring for five minutes more, or until the liquid has dried out and is absorbed.
- Slather unto burger buns. Best served Hot.

Baked Sriracha & Soy Sauce Tofu

Ingredients:

Extra-firm tofu- 1 block

Olive oil- ½ teaspoon

Mild soy sauce- 2 tablespoons

Sriracha- 1½ tablespoon

Directions:

- Prepare and preheat oven to 425F.
- Slice the tofu into bite sizes and shape of your choice. Quarter-sized squares are ideal while ensuring slices are about half an inch thick.
- In a mixing bowl, gently mix tofu, sriracha, olive oil, and soy sauce.
- Evenly spread mixture on a cookie sheet
- Bake at 425Ffor 10 minutes.
- Let settle for 10minutes, take out baking sheet from the oven then flip over each piece of tofu to bake the other side.
- Drizzle the leftover marinade on top of the tofu
- Bake at 425F for another 10-12 minutes.
- When the tofu has crispy texture outside, you can take it out from the oven.

Tofu Makhani

Ingredients:

For the marinated tofu:

Vegetable oil- 1 teaspoon

Extra-firm tofu- 1 block

Wrap the tofu block in a cheesecloth or paper napkin or cheesecloth, put it in a filter and put something heavy on it like a pan. Leave it like that for about an hour to sieve out the water. Then split it equally, and then slice it again in a cross like manner to give you four slices.

Coriander powder- 1 teaspoon

Red chilli powder- ¼ teaspoon

Turmeric- 1 teaspoon

Lemon juice- 1 tablespoon

Salt to taste

For the Makhani curry:

Oil- 1 tablespoon

3 green cardamom pods

3 cloves

10 peppercorns

Cinnamon- 1-inch piece

Cumin seeds- 1 tablespoon

Coriander powder- 1 tablespoon

Crushed garlic- ½ tablespoon

Crushed ginger- 1 tablespoon

Minced onion- 1 small

Finely diced tomato- 1 large

Tomato paste- ¼ cup

Turmeric- ½ teaspoon

Red chilli powder- ½ teaspoon

kasoori methi (dry fenugreek leaves)- 2 full tablespoons

Grated jaggery or maple syrup- 2 teaspoons (you can use sugar)

Vegetable broth- 2cups or more (you can use water but the broth gives it more spice)

Cashew nuts- ¼ cup

Vegan butter- 1 tablespoon

Lemon juice- 1 tablespoon

Fresh green coriander for garnish

Directions:
Preparation for the tofu:

- Combine ingredients except for the tofu.

- Slather the mixture marinade on the slices of tofu. Set aside to marinade for an hour.
- Evenly smear the oil on a cast-iron or nonstick griddle.
- Once griddle is hot, arrange the slices of tofu on it while avoiding crowding them.
- Allow to cook until tofu is golden-brown both sides, this takes around four minutes each side.
- Transfer to a plate and allow to cool.
- Once cool cut tofu into ¾-inch cubes. Set aside.
- To make the Makhani Curry:
- In a saucepan, heat the oil over medium heat.
- Add in the cumin seeds, and cook until they sputter.
- Add in peppercorns, cardamom, cinnamon, and cloves.
- Stir-fry for a minute over medium-high heat.
- Add in the onions and season with a little salt.
- Stir-fry until the onions begin to brown, around five minutes.

- Add in garlic and ginger pastes, kasoori methi, and cashew nuts.
- Stir-fry for another minute.
- Add in the tomato paste and tomatoes, turmeric, powdered coriander, and chili powder.
- Continue to cook the mixture while constantly stirring until the tomatoes become very soft and melt into the sauce.
- Should the mixture start to dry before the tomatoes are cooked, pour some water or vegetable stock and continue to cook until tomatoes are done.
- Once the tomatoes have softened, remove from the heat and allow the mixture to cool.
- Pour it into a blender and pour in a cup of vegetable stock.
- Blend mixture into a smooth paste. (avoid combining the mixture while hot as this would be dangerous. A hand blender is ideal for use)
- After mixing, transfer the paste back into the saucepan
- Cook again and add the left-over vegetable stock if the mixture is thick

- Bring it to a simmer and stir in the tofu cubes
- Season with salt to taste.
- Continue to simmer for about 10 minutes.
- Add in the vegan butter and remove from heat.
- Slowly stir to melt the butter and mix it into the sauce.
- Pour in lemon juice and maple syrup
- Stir and mix well
- Serve hot with some boiled rice or naan, with coriander leaves as garnish

Simple Vegan Tofu Lasagna

Ingredients:

Natural cooking spray oil

Filtered firm tofu- 1 package (14-ounce) package

Nutritional yeast- 2 tablespoons

Garlic granules- 1 teaspoon

Salt and pepper to taste

Vegan marinara sauce- 2 jars (25-ounce)

Cored, diced bell peppers- 3

Uncooked dried lasagna noodles- 12

Directions:
- Prepare and preheat oven to 350°F.
- Prepare a (9- x 13-inch) baking dish and lightly oil it. Set aside.
- Use paper towels to wrap tofu, about 3 or 4 layers, then gently press on tofu to get rid of as much water as possible. Chang the wrap, a couple of times as needed.
- Move tofu to a large bowl and add garlic, yeast, salt, and pepper and mash with a masher or the back of a fork. Set the mixture aside.
- In a medium pot, add marinara sauce and bring it to a simmer.
- Add in peppers and allow to simmering until they are tender just about 10 minutes.
- Scoop out enough marinara sauce into a separate dish to cover the bottom of the

lasagna and then arrange 4 pieces pasta on top.
- Spread about one-third of the tofu mixture on top of the pasta and then scoop up more sauce and spread it over the tofu.
- Repeat step 7 and 8 twice more, ending with the sauce on top.
- Cover the dish with foil and bake at 350°F until pasta is tender, about 45 to 60 minutes.
- Remove from the oven, set aside and allow to cool for 10 minutes and then serve.

Chapter 3: Smoothies

Coffee Cashew Smoothie

Ingredients:

Cashews soaked for 6 hours or all through the night in water - 1/4 cup

Peeled and diced banana - 1/2 banana (refrigerate if needed)

Cacao nibs - 1 tablespoon

Ice – ½ cup

Cold coffee - 1/4 cup

Unsweetened almond milk - 1 cup

Coconut sugar - 1/2 tablespoon (optional)

Directions:
- In a blender, place all and blend until smooth.

Raspberry Walnut Smoothie

Ingredients:
Refrigerated banana - 1/2

Walnuts - 1/4 cup

Unsweetened almond milk - 1 cup

Cacao nibs - 1 tablespoon

Vanilla - 1 teaspoon

Frozen raspberries - 1/3 cup

Instructions:
- In a blender, put all and blend until smooth.

Cinnamon Apple Smoothie

Ingredients:
Diced apple - 1 small

Rolled oats - 1/2 cup

Cinnamon - 1/2 teaspoon

Nutmeg - 1/2 teaspoon

Almond butter - 1 tablespoon

Unsweetened coconut milk - 1/2 cup

Ice cubes - 3-4

Chilled water - 1/2 cup

Directions:
- Place the oats and water in your blender.
- Pulse a couple of times to combine, then let it sit for a minimum of 2-3 minutes to allow the oats to soften.
- Mix all remaining ingredients to the oat mixture in the same blender.
- Blend all ingredients until smooth, about 30 seconds.
- Serve into a glass and sprinkle with a little bit of cinnamon and nutmeg.

Green Protein Power Breakfast Smoothie

Ingredients:

Unsweetened almond milk - 1 cup (250ml)

Ripe refrigerated banana - 1

Diced refrigerated mango - 1/2 cup (125 ml)

Young spinach - 2 large handfuls

Pumpkin seeds (Pepita seeds) - 1/4 cup (60ml)

Hemp hearts(hulled hemp seeds) - 2 tablespoons (30 ml)

Optional: 1/2 scoop vanilla protein powder and 1/4 cup water

Directions:
- You can use a blender or large tumbler in case you're using an immersion type blender
- Layer the banana, spinach, mango, hemp hearts, and pumpkin seeds inside the blender or tumbler.
- Pour in the almond milk and pulse until smooth.
- Some can use a cheap 15$ immersion blender and blend these ingredients for about 2 minutes (just enough time to blend the pumpkin seeds into a smooth consistency)
- This makes one serving of 16 oz.

Apple Spinach Protein Smoothie

Ingredients:

Organic apple - 1 large

Organic spinach - 3-4 cups

Organic almond butter - 1 tablespoon

Vega Sport vanilla protein powder - 1 scoop or pack

Unsweetened original almond milk - 1 cup

Ice cubes - 4-5

Directions:

• Combine all the ingredients except for the spinach in a blender and process until smooth.

• Put in spinach in batches, a handful per batch and blend it each time until all ingredients are incorporated.

• Pour mixture into a glass and serve.

Cofee Cashew and Cacao Protein Smoothie

Ingredients:

Diced and refrigerated organic banana, sliced and frozen - 1 large

Cold coffee - 1/2 cup

Organic fair trade cacao nibs - around 2 Tablespoons

Crushed hemp seeds - 2 Tablespoon

Unsweetened original almond milk - 1 cup

Cashews (20 nuts soaked for 6 hours in water) - 1/4 cup

Directions:
- Prepare coffee the night before. Brew it and then refrigerate.
- In a bowl, place raw cashews and submerge them in with water. Leave them to soak overnight.
- Combine all the ingredients in a blender and process until it is smooth.
- Serve in a glass and enjoy!

Protein Frosty Shake

Ingredients:

Daily Burn Fuel-6 in chocolate - 2 scoops

Unsweetened almond milk - 1 cup

1/2 banana

Ice - 2 cups

Xanthan gum - ½ teaspoon

Vanilla extract - ¼ teaspoon

Directions:
- In a blender, place all and blend until smooth.

Chocolate Peanut Butter Protein Shake

Ingredients:

Daily Burn Fuel-6 chocolate protein powder - 2 scoops

Unsweetened almond milk, soy milk or skim milk - 1 cup

1 banana

Peanut butter - 2 tablespoons

Ice cubes - 3-5 cubes

Directions:
- In a blender, place all and blend until smooth.

Cherry Almond Smoothie

Ingredients:

Pitted fresh or frozen cherries - 1 cup

Vanilla protein powder - 1 scoop

Almond butter - 2 teaspoons

Pure almond extract - 1 teaspoon

Maca root powder - 1/2 teaspoon (optional) it has no effect on the taste or shape

Camu camu powder - 1/2 teaspoon (a very strong food that contains numerous amounts of anti-inflammatory and anti-oxidant properties (optional)

Water or unsweetened almond milk - 1 cup

Ice cubes - 6-8 cubes

Guar gum - 1/2 teaspoon for creamy taste (optional)

Directions:
- In a blender, combine all ingredients except for the ice and guar gum.
- Process until mixture is almost smooth.
- Add in guar gum and ice, and continue to process.
- Pour into glasses and serve.

Blueberry Banana Protein Smoothie

Ingredients:
Fresh or frozen blueberries - 1 cup

Soft ripe bananas - 1 (you can refrigerate some)

Water/coconut water - 1 cup for additional sweetness

Vanilla extract - 1 teaspoon

Chia seeds - 2 tablespoons

Lemon - 1 zest

Optional

1 serving soy vanilla protein powder for extra protein

Directions:
- Combine all the ingredients in a blender, and add in lemon zest grated from a fresh lemon.
- Blend until mixture is smooth.

Cinnamon Apple Smoothie

Ingredients:
Diced apple - 1 small

Rolled oats - 1/2 cup

Cinnamon - 1/2 teaspoon

Nutmeg - 1/2 teaspoon

Almond butter - 1 tablespoon

Unsweetened coconut milk - 1/2 cup

Ice cubes - 3-4

Chilled water - 1/2 cup

Directions:

- Place all ingredients in a blender, and pulse for about 10-15 seconds.
- If you want to consume it immediately, add three ice cubes to cool it.
- If you are preparing this ahead of time as a reserve, refrigerate overnight before serving.

Chapter 4: Snacks

Blueberry Lemon Protein Scones

Ingredients:

Pure all-purpose flour- 1½ cups and extra for dusting

Whole white wheat or whole-grain pastry flour- 1 cup

Baking powder- 1 tablespoon

Baking soda- 1 teaspoon

Salt- ½ teaspoon

Nearly iced refined coconut oil- ¼ cup

Near frozen canola oil- ¼ cup canola oil (sounds strange freezing canola oil)

Unsweetened, plain soy/almond milk- 1 cup

Brown rice protein powder- ½ cup

Organic sugar- 1cup and extra for spraying

Freshly juiced lemon- 3 tablespoons

Pure vanilla extract- 1 teaspoon

Crushed lemon- 1 zest

Iced blueberries- 1 cup (kept frozen)

Canola oil for brushing

*Mix canola and coconut oil in a small plastic container and refrigerate it for 20–25 minutes, or until it thickens. The oil should look like ice or frozen milk. Leave to defrost for about 5 minutes if it is too iced.

Directions:

• Transfer coconut and canola oil into a small plastic container then refrigerate for 20–25 minutes, or until the oil becomes very thick and cloudy.

• The oils should have sorbet like consistency. If it is too hard or tough, you can just leave outside the fridge for about 5 minutes to defrost until it softens.

• Prepare and preheat the oven to 400°F.

• Then cover a baking sheet with parchment paper.

• Meanwhile, in a big bowl, combine dry ingredients: the flours, baking soda, the baking powder, and salt.

• In the center of the mixture, form a well.

- Using a blender, blend the almost frozen oils, rice protein powder, soy/almond milk, lemon juice, organic sugar, vanilla, and lemon zest until it has a smooth consistency.
- Pour the blended mixture into the center of the dry ingredients, the flour well you formed.
- Add the frozen blueberries.
- Stir and mix just enough to create a dough that is soft. Avoid overmixing the dough.
- Prepare your work space for the scones by dusting your work surface with some flour
- Transfer the dough onto this workspace.
- Cut the dough in half and form half into a disk shape just less than an inch thick.
- Cut and divide each disk into six wedges.
- Relocate the wedges onto the parchment paper.
- Brush the wedges with canola oil on top and sprinkle it with sugar.
- Bake at 400°F for 20–22 minutes, or just until the wedges turn a light brown color and are firm.

- Serve them warm, or you can have them split and toasted on a pan.

Loaded Blueberry Muffins

Ingredients:

wet ingredients

cup olive oil - 1/2

dry ingredients

buckwheat flour - 2 cups

brown rice flour - 1 cup

potato starch - 1/2 cup

xanthan gum – 1 tsp

baking soda - 1 tsp

baking powder - 1 1/2 tsp

sea salt - 1 tsp

2 tbsp flaxseed meal mixed with 4 tbsp water

organic granulated sugar - 3/4 cup

shredded zucchini (about 1 medium) - 1 1/3 cups

2 smashed medium ripe bananas

vanilla extract - 1 tsp

fresh blueberries - 1 cup

Directions:
- Prepare and preheat oven to 350 °F.
- Prepare two standard sized muffin pans and line cups with paper liners.
- In a big bowl, combine all wet ingredients and mix well.
- Meanwhile, In a separate bowl, use a whisk to combine all waterless ingredients.
- Progressively add in the dry ingredients to the wet ingredients until they are thoroughly combined. The batter will have a thick consistency.
- Pour about 1/4 cup batter into each muffin cup then lightly sprinkle with brown sugar.
- Bake 350 °F for 25 minutes, or until you see the tops have formed are have turned a light golden brown color.
- Allow to cool for a few minutes before serving.

Petite Vanilla Bean Scones

Ingredients:

Makes around 20 mini scones

unbleached all-purpose flour – 2 cup

baking powder - 1 1/2 tsp

salt - 1/4 tsp

vegan butter, butter (used Earth Balance Organic Coconut Spread) - 1/2 cup

sugar - 1/3 cup

1 vanilla bean

non dairy milk - 1/2 cup

Vanilla Bean Glaze

confectioners' sugar - 1 cup

Coconut or Vegan Creamer - 2 Tbsp

Directions:

- Prepare and preheat oven to 400F.
- In a medium bowl, use a whisk to mix dry ingredients: flour, baking powder, salt, and sugar.
- Slice a vanilla bean in half lengthwise then scrape seeds out using a small, sharp knife and drop it into the dry mixture.

- With a couple of knives or a pastry blender or, slice the butter spread and add into the flour mixture
- Mix until ingredients are well combined, showing no remaining chunks of coconut spread/butter.
- Using a wooden spoon or spatula, mix in milk and stir.
- The dough will still be dry, however, if you are not able to incorporate all the dry ingredients add a tablespoon more milk. The dough should not be wet.
- From the dough, make 5 equal balls and flatten each to form a disc of about 1/2 – 3/4-inch thick.
- Divide each disk into quarters then arrange them on a non-stick cookie/baking sheet or you can opt to line a baking sheet with a parchment paper or Silpat mat.
- Bake at 400F for 12-14 minutes, until their edges turn a light golden color.
- Allow to cool on a wire rack before your start glazing.
- In a big bowl, use a whisk to combine sugar and creamer/milk.

- Add in any vanilla bean seeds that are left over from the recipe (scrape the same vanilla pod a second time or use half a section from another bean).
- Pour the mixture over the cooled scones for a glaze. Enjoy!

Conclusion

More and more people are adopting the vegan lifestyle, and it certainly does not mean you have to to sacrifice your fitness or muscle building goals. Vegetable protein diets can be constructed effectively for athletes and bodybuilders, as many have established. Consideration of details is vital for total energy, protein, essential fats, vitamin B12 and minerals like iron, calcium and zinc. I hope the readers of this recipe book will be convinced of the benefits of a vegan diet and also learn of the importance of protein in your daily diet, rich sources of vegetarian protein and even non-vegans can enjoy these scrumptious protein bars.

Part 2

Introduction

This vegan dessert cookbook includes a variety of unique and delicious cake, cookie and dessert recipes that you can easily make at home. As a professional vegan baker I have come across all kinds of vegan dessert recipes, and I would like to share my favorite dessert recipes with you. I have provided easy to follow steps in these recipes, so both beginner and novice vegan bakers can make these recipes.

These recipes were the most popular in my bakery, and I think you will really enjoy them!

Lemon Squares

Ingredients

Crust:

1 cup all-purpose flour

5 tablespoons margarine

1/4 cup granulated sugar

Filling:

3 egg replacers

3/4 cup granulated sugar

3 tablespoons all-purpose flour

1 teaspoon real vanilla

1/2 teaspoon baking powder

1/8 teaspoon salt

2 lemons, zested and juiced

powdered sugar, optional

Directions

Preheat oven to 350 degrees F.

To make crust:

In a bowl, combine crust ingredients and press into 8 X 8 inch pan. Bake for 15 minutes.

To make filling:

While crust is baking, beat the egg replacers in a bowl until foamy. Add the remainder of the filling ingredients and mix together. Pour over the crust, and bake 20 minutes, or until set.

Let cool before serving.

Key Lime Pie

Ingredients

2 8 oz. containers vegan cream cheese

2 tablespoon soy milk

1 cup natural sugar

1 teaspoon vanilla

2 teaspoon grated lime peel

4 tablespoon lime juice

2 tablespoon cornstarch

1 - 9inch vegan graham cracker crust

Sliced strawberries

Directions

Preheat oven to 350 degrees. Blend cream cheese, soymilk, vegan sugar, vanilla, grated lime peel, lime juice and cornstarch until smooth.

Pour mixture into graham cracker crust, place on baking sheet and bake for 40 minutes.

Let cool, and refrigerate 4 hours. Top with sliced strawberries.

Vegan Cheesecake

Ingredients

Crust:

18 vegan graham crackers or other cookies, crumbled

1/2 cup canola oil

1 tablespoon all-purpose flour

1 tablespoon agave or maple syrup

Filling:

1 (10-ounce or 300 g) package silken tofu, pressed lightly to remove water

2/3 cup raw cashews, soaked overnight and drained

1 tablespoon lemon juice

2 teaspoons canola oil

1/3 cup raw sugar or other sweetener

3-1/2 teaspoons Egg Replacer (no water added)

1/2 teaspoon vanilla extract

1/2 teaspoon salt

Directions

To make crust:

Combine all crust ingredients in a large bowl. Mix until well incorporated, and then press into pie dish.

To make filling:

Combine soaked cashews, silken tofu, canola oil, and lemon juice in a blender; pulse until completely smooth and creamy.

Transfer mixture to a bowl and whisk in sugar, egg replacer, vanilla, and salt until completely dissolved, making sure there are no lumps or sugar crystals. Carefully spoon mixture into the crust.

Bake at 375 F for 25 to 30 minutes, until set. Remove from oven and let cool.

Place in fridge for at least five hours to chill.

Vegan Chocolate Fudge Brownies

Ingredients

1/4 cup canola oil

1/3 cup water

1 cup organic sugar

1 cup organic unbleached flour

1 tablespoon ground flax seed

1/3 cup unsweetened cocoa powder

1/2 teaspoon baking powder

1/4 teaspoon salt

Directions

Preheat oven to 350 F. Mix wet ingredients in large bowl, then add in all the dry ingredients and mix. Do not over mix.

Place in oven and bake for 20-25 minutes.

Chocolate Vegan Cheesecake

Ingredients

1 (12 ounce) package silken tofu

1 (8 ounce) tub vegan cream cheese

3/4 cup sugar

1 (12 ounce) package vegan chocolate chips

3 tablespoons maple syrup

1 (9") vegan graham cracker pie crust

Directions

In blender, blend tofu until smooth. With an electric mixer in medium bowl, combine vegan sugar and cream cheese and 2 tablespoons of the smoothed tofu, and beat until smooth.

Add cream cheese mixture to blender with remaining tofu. Blend again until smooth.

Melt chocolate chips in double boiler, or microwave. Add melted chips to blender, blend until chocolate is mixed, this may require some stirring. After chips and mixture are well blended, add maple syrup, blend for 30 seconds.

Pour mixture into pie crust until full, and refrigerate until set.

Chocolate Banana Cake

Ingredients

2 very ripe medium bananas

1 1/4 cups all-purpose white, unbleached flour

3/4 cup sugar (half white and half brown)

1/4 cup unsweetened cocoa powder

1/3 cup canola oil

1/3 cup water

1 teaspoon baking soda

1 teaspoon white vinegar

1/4 teaspoon salt

1/3 cup vegan semisweet chocolate chips

Directions

Preheat oven to 350F. Mash bananas or blend with electric beater.

Blend in wet ingredients and brown sugar. Sift dry ingredients together then add to wet.

Blend well then pour into a greased 8X8 square cake pan. Sprinkle chocolate chips over batter.

Bake about 35 minutes or until toothpick inserted in the center comes out clean. Cool completely before serving.

Creamy Peanut Butter Pie

Ingredients

Filling:

4 squares of unsweetened bakers chocolate

2/3 cup peanut butter

16-18oz silken tofu

1 cup sugar

4-6 tablespoon soy milk

Vegan graham cracker crust

Directions

Melt the chocolate and blend with the tofu, peanut butter, and sugar adding soy milk to the desired texture.

Pour filling into the graham cracker pie crust and refrigerate.

Strawberry Cheesecake

Ingredients

2 (8 ounce) containers vegan cream cheese

1 cup unrefined sugar

2 teaspoons vanilla

3 tablespoons lemon juice

2 tablespoons cornstarch

1 vegan graham cracker crust

1/2-3/4 pound fresh strawberries, halved lengthwise

Directions

Preheat oven to 350 F. Combine cream cheese, sugar, and vanilla in a food processor or blender. Add lemon juice and blend some more.

Once finished blending add the cornstarch. Pour mixture into the crust and bake for 45 minutes.

Let cool before serving, and once completely cooled, add strawberries on top.

Lemon Bundt Cake

Ingredients

1 and 2/3 cups granulated sugar

2/3 cups canola oil

1 14 oz can of lite coconut milk

1/4 cup of rice milk

1/4 cup lemon juice

3 tablespoons finely grated lemon zest

2 teaspoons vanilla extract

3 cup whole wheat pastry flour

2 teaspoons baking powder

1 teaspoons baking soda

1 teaspoons salt

1/2 cup shredded unsweetened coconut

Directions

Preheat the oven to 350F . Lightly grease an 8 x10 inch bundt pan.

In a large mixing bowl, combine the granulated sugar, oil, coconut milk, rice, soy or almond milk, lemon juice and zest and vanilla. Stir to combine.

Sift the flour, baking powder, baking soda, and salt into the wet ingredients in batches, mixing well after each addition. Fold in the coconut.

Pour the batter into the Bundt pan. Bake for 1 hour, or until a knife inserted through the cake comes out clean. Remove from the oven and let cool for about 10 minutes, then place a cutting board over the cake pan, gently flip over, and release the cake from the pan.

Let cool completely. Once cooled, you can option to sift a sprinkling of confectioner's sugar over the top. Slice and serve.

Cranberry Banana Cookies

Ingredients

1 banana

1 cup soft margarine

1/2 cup white sugar

1/2 cup packed brown sugar

1 teaspoon vanilla

1.5 cups flour

1 teaspoon baking soda

1 teaspoon cinnamon

1 teaspoon ground nutmeg

3 cups oatmeal

1/2 cup dried cranberries

1/2 cup sliced almonds

Directions

Preheat over to 350F. Mash banana with a fork, then mix with margarine, sugars, and vanilla in a bowl until smooth.

In a separate bowl, mix the flour, baking soda, cinnamon, and nutmeg. Mix the wet with the dry, then add oatmeal, cranberries, and almonds.

Spoon onto a ungreased cookie sheet, and bake for about 15 minutes. Let cool and serve.

Vegan Vanilla Cake

Ingredients

1 1/2 cups flour

1 cup sugar

1/2 teaspoon baking soda

1/2 teaspoon salt

1 cup ice cold water

1/2 cup oil

2 teaspoons vanilla

2 tablespoons lemon juice

Directions

Preheat oven to 375 F. Grease an 8" or 9" cake pan. In a bowl, sift together flour, sugar, baking soda and salt until very fine.

In a small bowl, combine cold water, oil, and vanilla. Add liquid ingredients (except lemon juice) to dry and combine. Once the batter is combined, add the lemon juice and stir quickly then pour into prepared pan.

Bake for 25 to 30 minutes or until toothpick comes out clean.

Chocolate Chip Cookies

Ingredients

2 cups all purpose flour

2 teaspoons baking powder

1/2 teaspoons sea salt

2 teaspoons cinnamon

1 cup sugar

1/2 cup canola oil

1 teaspoons vanilla

1/2 cup water

1 cup vegan chocolate chips

Directions

Preheat oven to 350 F.

Mix all ingredients together in a large bowl, until well combined.

Using a small scoop, place mixture on a lightly greased cookie sheet.

Bake 10-12 minutes. (Note: Cookies won't brown on top when done.)

Carrot Cake

Ingredients

1 1/2 cup self rising flour

1 cup raw sugar

1 teaspoon baking soda

1 teaspoon cinnamon

1/4 teaspoon salt

1 cup of shredded carrots

3/4 cup orange juice

1/3 cup grapeseed oil

1 teaspoon vanilla

1 tablespoon ground flax seed

Directions

Heat oven to 350F. Mix all dry ingredients in bowl. then add carrots. Stir until well coated. Add remaining wet ingredients and stir just until blended. Pour into ungreased 9 inch square non stick pan.

Bake 25-30 minutes. Let cool before serving.

Applesauce Cranberry Cake

Ingredients

2 cups applesauce, unsweetened

1 cup granulated sugar

1/2 cup apple juice, unsweetened

1/4 cup mild olive oil

2 teaspoons flax seed meal (ground flax)

1 teaspoon vanilla

1 1/4 cups whole wheat flour

1 1/2 cups white flour

1 teaspoon cinnamon

1/4 teaspoon cloves

1/4 teaspoon ginger

2 teaspoon baking powder

3/4 teaspoon salt

1/2 cup walnuts, chopped

1/2 cup dried cranberries

Directions

Preheat oven to 350 degrees. Spray a 9 X 13 inch baking pan with nonstick spray.

In a large mixing bowl combine the applesauce, sugar, apple juice, olive oil, flax meal and vanilla. Stir till thoroughly combined.

In another bowl combine the whole wheat and white flours, spices, walnuts and raisins or cranberries. Gently add to the wet ingredients and stir just until combined.

Pour into pan and bake for 35 to 40 minutes until a toothpick inserted in the center comes out clean. Remove from pan when cool.

Oatmeal Cookies

Ingredients

1/3 cup silken soft tofu

1/3 cup vegetable/canola oil

1/4 cup apple juice or concentrate

1 tablespoon vanilla extract

1/2 cup raw vegan sugar

1/4 cup maple syrup

2 cup quick oats

2 cup flour

1/2 teaspoon baking powder and 1/2 teaspoon baking soda

1/2 teaspoon salt

2 cup vegan chocolate chips or carob chips

1 cup walnuts

Directions

In a medium-sized bowl, blend flour, baking soda, salt, and baking powder. In a separate bowl, whip tofu with a mixer until creamy. Add oil, apple juice, vanilla, vegan sugar at low speed mix until vegan sugar is somewhat dissolved.

Add vegan maple syrup and mix 1 minute. Add oats and flour mixture, blend for 2 more minutes or until well blended. Then fold in walnuts and chocolate chips.

Drop large tablespoons of dough on well oiled cookie sheet. Slightly flatten with back of spoon and bake 13-15 minutes at 350 F.

Peanut Butter Cookies

Ingredients

3 tablespoons egg replacer + 4 tablespoons water

2 1/4 cups unbleached whole wheat flour

1 1/4 cup natural crunchy peanut butter

2/3 cup maple syrup

1/2 cup Sucanat

1/2 cup margarine

1/2 tablespoon baking powder

Directions

Preheat oven to 350 F. Mix egg replacer and water. In large bowl, combine all ingredients, and mix.

Roll tablespoons of dough into balls, and place 2" apart on cookie sheet. Flatten balls with flour dipped fork, in criss-cross pattern.

Bake 15 minutes or until lightly browned.

Apple Cake

Ingredients

1 cup flour

1 cup semolina

1 cup sugar

1 teaspoon baking powder

1 cup vegan margarine, melted

5 large or 8-10 small apples

Directions

Preheat oven to 375F degrees.

Mix flour, sugar, semolina and baking powder in a bowl. Peel and grate the apples in a separate bowl, and melt the margarine.

Spray a baking dish with cooking spray or rub with margarine. Spread a third of the dry mixture, cover with a third of the apples, repeating.

Pour melted margarine on top, and bake for 1 hour.

Coconut Lemon Cake

Ingredients

20 oz sugar

8 oz non-hydrogenated margarine

¼ cup lemon juice

grated zest of 4 lemons

2 teaspoons vanilla

1 ½ tablespoons lemon extract

24.6 oz flour

2 tablespoons baking powder

1 ½ teaspoons baking soda

1 ½ teaspoons salt

2 cups water

2 cups premium coconut milk

Filling

¾ - 1 cup pure raspberry jam, warmed slightly until spreadable

1/3 cup fine-shred coconut

Directions

Preheat oven to 350F, grease 2 9x13 pans.

Cream together sugar and margarine. Add lemon juice, zest, vanilla and lemon extracts and beat well. Whisk together dry ingredients in a medium bowl.

Add dry ingredients in three sections, alternating with the water and coconut milk. Beat well after each addition. Divide between pans and bake 45 minutes, or until cake tests done.

Cool completely in the pan before turning out onto a tray, then chill 1 hour before filling. Spread jam evenly over one of the layers and sprinkle with coconut.

Place second layer on top, trim the edges and chill again before frosting and decorating.

Chocolate Chip Pumpkin Cookies

Ingredients

1 cup vegetable oil

4 cup sugar

2 egg substitute (flax seeds and water works well)

5 cups flour

1/4 teaspoon ground ginger

2 teaspoons baking powder

2 teaspoons baking soda

2 teaspoons nutmeg

2 teaspoons cinnamon

1 teaspoon all-spice

1 3/4 teaspoons salt

1 29 oz. can of pumpkin

2 cup vegan chocolate chips

1 cup chopped walnuts

Directions

Beat oil and vegan sugar in mixing bowl. Add egg substitutes and beat well.

In a separate bowl, stir together the flour, baking powder, baking soda, spices, and salt.

Add vegan sugar mixture alternatively with pumpkin into flour mixture. Stir well after each addition. Fold in chocolate chips, walnuts, and vanilla.

Drop by teaspoon onto a greased cookie sheet. Bake for 15-20 minutes or until golden brown at 350 F.

Pumpkin Cheesecake

Ingredients

5 (8 oz.) packages vegan cream cheese

½ cup silken tofu

½ cup soy creamer

¾ cup maple syrup

3 tablespoons egg substitute powder

3 tablespoons flour

2 teaspoons ground cinnamon

1 teaspoon ground ginger

1 teaspoon ground cloves

1 tablespoon vanilla extract

1 can pumpkin (15 oz.)

1 ½ cup fine graham cracker crumbs

6 tablespoons melted margarine

1/4 cup sugar

Directions

Preheat oven to 350 F.

For the crust: Mix the crumbs, vegan margarine and vegan sugar together well and press into greased 10" spring form pan. Bake crust for 10 minutes, take out and let cool. Raise oven temperature to 425 degrees.

Beat together the egg substitute and vegan maple syrup.

In a large bowl, beat together cream vegan cheese, silken tofu, soy creamer, vegan sugar, and egg substitute mixture. Add the flour and spices, then the vanilla. Add the pumpkin and beat at medium speed until well blended.

Pour the mixture into the prepared crust and bake for 15 minutes. Reduce the temperature to 275 F and bake for an additional hour. Turn off the heat but leave the cake in the oven to cool for several hours or overnight.

Serve the cake either warm or chilled, with whipped tofu.

Gingersnap Cookies

Ingredients

4 tablespoons margarine

1/2 cup raw sugar

Egg replacer equivalent to 1 egg

2 1/2 cups plain flour

1 teaspoon bicarbonate of soda

4 teaspoon ground ginger

1 teaspoon ground cloves

2 teaspoon ground cinnamon

2 teaspoon ground nutmeg

3 tablespoons golden syrup

Directions

Preheat oven to 350F.

Cream margarine and raw sugar, add egg replacement, mix. Add flour, soda and spices, then golden syrup and mix well.

Roll mixture into teaspoon sized balls, flatten slightly and place on cookie tray.

Bake for 10 minutes in at 350F.

Green Tea Cookies

Ingredients

½ cup vegan butter spread

½ cup unrefined coconut oil (not refined)

2 tablespoons matcha green tea powder

¼ cup + ½ cup powdered sugar, divided

¼ cup sweetened shredded coconut (optional)

2¼ cups all-purpose flour

Directions

Preheat oven to 400º F.

Cream together buttery spread, coconut oil, green tea powder and ¼ cup powdered sugar until smooth. Add shredded coconut and flour and mix until combined. Mixture will be somewhat crumbly but should stick together.

Roll dough into 24 balls, approximately 1½ inches in size. Place on an ungreased cookie sheet and bake in preheated oven for 10-12 minutes or just until set.

Place ½ cup powdered sugar in a wide, shallow dish; set aside.

Remove cookies from oven and allow to cool for 10-15 minutes. Roll each cookie in powdered sugar and set aside until completely cooled.

Peanut Butter Balls

Ingredients

3/4 cup raw pumpkin seeds

3/4 cup raw sunflower seeds

1/2 cup pitted dates

1/2 cup peanut butter

1 tablespoon chia seeds

Directions

Blend together all ingredients, using a food processor.

Roll into balls and chill in refrigerator.

Banana Cake

Ingredients

1/4 cup margarine

3/4 cup sugar

2 bananas, mashed

1 teaspoon vanilla extract

3/4 cup soy milk

3/4 cup rice flour

1/2 cup potato starch

3 teaspoons baking powder

1 teaspoons xanthan gum

pinch of salt

4 teaspoons powdered egg replacer

1/4 cup carob powder

Directions

Set oven to 375°F. Grease and line cake tin.

Cream vegan margarine and vegan sugar. Beat in bananas and vanilla.

Sift together flours, baking powder, salt, xanthan gum, egg replacer powder, and carob powder.

Add soy milk and sifted dry ingredients alternatively, one-third at a time, mixing lightly.

Place mixture in cake tin and bake at 375°F for 35 minutes.

Cake is cooked when a skewer placed into the centre of the cake comes out clean.

Let cake cool before serving. Sprinkle with vegan icing or confectioners sugar.

Apple Spice Cookies

Ingredients

1 cup flour

- 1 cup brown sugar
- 1/2 cup white sugar
- 3 cups oats
- 1 teaspoon baking soda
- 1 teaspoon cinnamon
- 1/2 teaspoon nutmeg
- 1/2 teaspoon ginger
- 1/2 teaspoon cloves
- 1/2 cup almond milk
- 1/2 cup vegetable oil
- 1 teaspoon vanilla extract
- 2 small apples, unpeeled and diced

Directions

Preheat oven to 350 F and line 2 large cookie sheets with parchment paper. Mix all dry ingredients.

Make a well in center, and add wet ingredients. Knead with hands until mixture is moist, while stirring in apples.

Drop large spoonfuls of mixture on sheets. Bake for 15-18 minutes.

Easy Date Banana Cookies

Ingredients

36 dates

1 1/2 cups water or soymilk

1/4 - ½ cups sugar

2 cups flour

1/2 cup oil

2 teaspoons baking soda

3 bananas

Directions

Preheat oven to 350 F and oil an 8x8 inch metal baking pan.

Put dates, soymilk/water, sugar and bananas in a blender or food processor and blend/process until dates are pureed and well combined.

Pour date mixture in a large bowl and add the oil. Stir well to incorporate. Add flour slowly, then baking soda.

When you have incorporated all of the flour into the batter, pour into the baking pan and bake for 60 minutes or until toothpick test comes out clean, check after 40 minutes for doneness.

Spice Cake

Ingredients

3 cups flour

2 cups sugar

2 bags of chai tea

2 teaspoons baking soda

1 teaspoon salt

2 cups water

1/3 cup olive or vegetable oil

2 teaspoons vanilla

2 teaspoons cinnamon

2 tablespoons vinegar

Directions

Preheat oven to 350F.

Cut open the bags of chai tea and pour out the spices. In a bowl add the dry ingredients together and stir. Then add the water, oil and vanilla. Add the vinegar in last mixing in well, and pour mixture into cake pan.

Bake at 350F for 40 minute to an hour, or until toothpick comes out clean.

Oatmeal Raisin Cookies

Ingredients

1 1/2 cups firmly packed brown sugar

1 cup margarine

Egg replacer equivalent to 2 eggs

2 teaspoons water

2 teaspoons vanilla extract

2 cups all purpose flour

1 teaspoon baking powder

1 teaspoon baking soda

2 teaspoons ground cinnamon

1/2 teaspoon salt

2 cups quick-cooking oats, uncooked

1 cup raisins

Directions

Preheat oven to 350 F. Combine brown sugar and margarine in bowl and mix with spoon. Add egg replacer, water and vanilla, and continue mixing.

Add all remaining ingredients except oats and raisins. Mix well. Stir in oats and raisins.

Drop dough by rounded tablespoonfuls, 2 inches apart, onto cookie sheets. Bake 9-11 minutes or until lightly browned. Let stand 1 minute. Remove from cookie sheets, cool completely before serving.

Vegan Lemon Cookies

Ingredients

2 cups flour

2 teaspoons baking powder

1/4 teaspoon salt

grated rind of one lemon

1 cup sugar

1/2 cup vegetable oil

1/4 cup fresh lemon juice

Directions

Oil and flour a 9x9 inch pan. Preheat the oven to 350°F.

In a bowl, combine the flour, baking powder, salt, and grated lemon rind.

In a separate bowl, combine vegan sugar and oil. Add the lemon juice and mix well. Add the wet ingredients to the dry. Stir well. It makes a thick batter.

Spread the batter in the pan.

Bake for 30 minutes. Allow to cool and then cut into squares or bars.

Pecan Cheesecake

Ingredients

Crust:

1/4 cup pecans (chopped)

3 tablespoon raw sugar

1 1/2 cup vanilla wafers or vegan graham crackers

1/4 cup margarine (melted)

Filling:

1 pound vegan cream cheese

1 1/4 cup sugar

2 tablespoon pastry flour

3 tablespoon applesauce

1 1/2 teaspoon vanilla

1/2 cup pecans (chopped)

Directions

Crust:

Blend all ingredients except margarine. In mixing bowl, add wafer mixture and melted margarine to moisten. Place mixture in round foil pie pan, pressing down to cover the whole pan.

Bake at 350 F for 6 minutes. Remove from oven.

Filling:

Mix vegan cream cheese and sugar in bowl. Stir in flour, slowly add applesauce. Stir in vanilla and pecans.

Mix all ingredients well. Pour mixture onto wafer crust and bake at 350 F for 1 hour. Garnish top of cheesecake with pecan halves.

Coconut Banana Cookies

Ingredients

2 bananas, mashed

1 teaspoon vanilla extract

1/2 cup sugar

1/2 cup vegetable oil

3 teaspoons soy milk

1 cup flour

1 teaspoon baking soda

1 teaspoon cinnamon

1 cup rolled oats

1 cup shredded coconut

Directions

Preheat oven to 350 degrees F and lightly oil a cookie sheet. In blender/food processor, blend together mashed bananas, vanilla, sugar, oil, and milk.

In large bowl, sift together flour, baking soda, and cinnamon. Stir in the oats and then fold in the banana mixture well.

Fold in shredded coconut. Scoop spoon-sized portions onto prepared cookie sheet and bake for 15-20 minutes.

Lemon Cake

Ingredients

1 3/4 cups flour

1 teaspoon baking powder

1/2 teaspoon salt

1 large lemon

1/2 cup margarine (melted)

1 cup brown sugar

2 egg substitutes

2/3 cup soy milk

1/2 teaspoon vanilla

1/4 cup powdered sugar

Directions

Preheat oven to 350F.

Mix dry ingredients (except sugars). Finely grate lemon peel and stir it in. For the glaze, squeeze the lemons juice into a small bowl, mix with powdered sugar, and set aside.

Beat margarine and brown sugar together, add egg replacers, and add flour and soy milk. Add vanilla and mix well. Pour into a greased loaf pan and bake at 350F for an hour.

Let cool for at least 20 minutes, turn out onto a cooling rack, and drizzle with glaze.

Frosted Raspberry Chocolate Cake

Ingredients

1 1/2 cups flour

1/3 cup unsweetened cacao powder

1/2 teaspoon baking soda

1/2 teaspoon sea salt

1 cup brown sugar

1/2 cup grapeseed oil

1 cup chilled brewed coffee

2 teaspoons vanilla extract

2 tablespoons apple cider vinegar

Chocolate Raspberry Frosting

2 ounces unsweetened dark chocolate

1/4 cup fresh raspberries, mashed

3 tablespoons water

1 teaspoon vanilla extract

1 cup confectioners' (icing) sugar

Topping over frosting

1 cup fresh raspberries

½ cup non-dairy chocolate chips

Directions

Preheat oven to 375°F. Spread coconut oil on baking dish to prevent sticking.

Sift flour, cacao, baking soda, salt and sugar. In another bowl, combine oil, coffee and vanilla. Pour liquid into dry, and mix until smooth.

Add vinegar and stir briefly; baking soda will begin to react with vinegar. Quickly pour batter into prepared pan.

Bake for 25 to 30 minutes. Allow cake to cool slightly before adding frosting.

Frosting:

In heavy saucepan, melt chocolate over low to medium heat. Once fully melted, remove from heat and stir in mashed raspberries, water and vanilla. Stir in confectioners' sugar. Spread frosting on cooled cake.

Top frosting with whole raspberries and sprinkle non-dairy chocolate chips over cake.

Molasses Cookies

Ingredients

3/4 cup flour

1/2 cup sugar

2 cups oats

1/2 teaspoon baking soda

1/2 teaspoon baking powder

1/2 teaspoon salt

1/3 cup applesauce

1/4 cup maple syrup

1/4 cup molasses

1 tablespoon vanilla

Egg replacer equivalent to 1 egg

1 - 1 1/2 cups chopped dried apricots

1/2 cup shredded coconut

1 tablespoon vegetable oil

Directions

Preheat oven to 350 F. Combine the flour, oats, sugar, baking soda, baking powder, and salt. Mix well.

In a separate bowl, combine the applesauce, syrup, molasses, vanilla, and egg replace. Add a tablespoon of oil.

Combine the wet and dry ingredients and add the apricots and coconut as well.

Drop spoonfuls onto a greased cookie sheet, flattening out slightly. Bake 15-20 minutes until firm.

About the Author

Alton Hill is author of several cookbooks on Vegan diet. He has written research papers on the topic and currently lives in California.

www.ingramcontent.com/pod-product-compliance
Lightning Source LLC
LaVergne TN
LVHW011943070526
838202LV00054B/4782